30 MINUTE HEART HEALTHY COOKBOOK FOR SENIORS

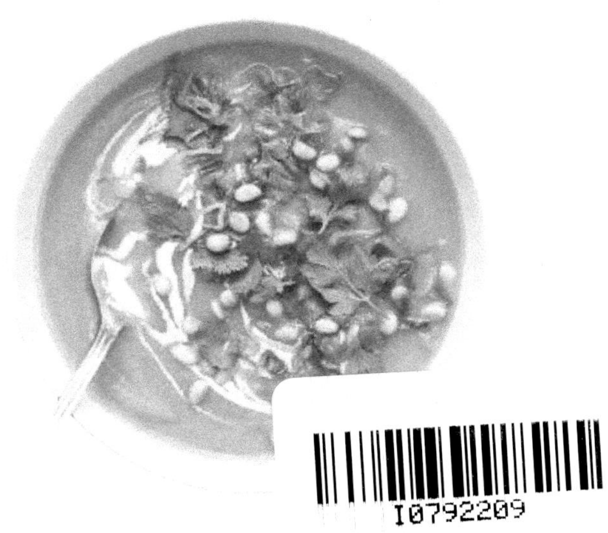

Low Fat Low Cholesterol Diet Recipes a Healthy Heart

Linda Carlucci

Copyright © 2024 by Linda Carlucci

DISCLAIMER

This cookbook is intended to provide general information and recipes.

The recipes provided in this cookbook are not intended to replace or be a substitute for medical advice from a physician.

The reader should consult a healthcare professional for any specific medical advice, diagnosis or treatment.

Any specific dietary advice provided in this cookbook is not intended to replace or be a substitute for medical advice from a physician.

The author is not responsible or liable for any adverse effects experienced by readers of this cookbook as a result of following the recipes or dietary advice provided.

The author makes no representations or warranties of any kind (express or implied) as to the accuracy, completeness, reliability or suitability of the recipes provided in this cookbook.

The author disclaims any and all liability for any damages arising out of the use or misuse of the recipes provided in this cookbook. The reader must also take care to ensure that the recipes provided in this cookbook are prepared and cooked safely.

The recipes provided in this cookbook are for informational purposes only and should not be used as a substitute for professional medical advice, diagnosis or treatment.

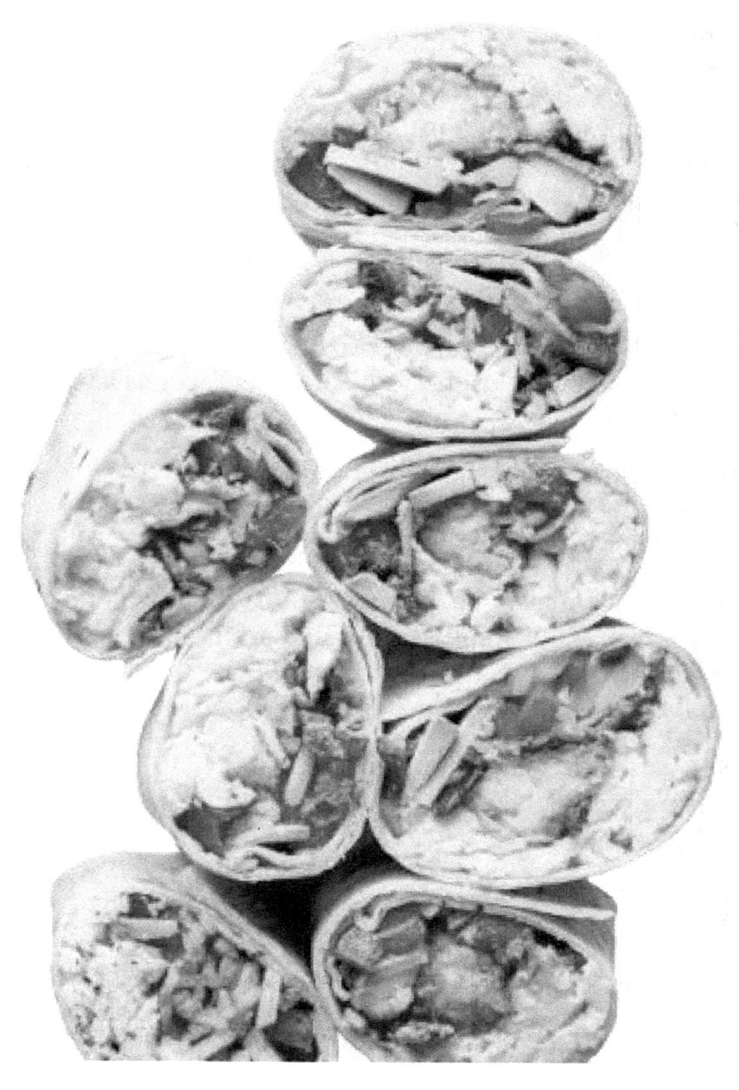

TABLE OF CONTENTS

INTRODUCTION

A heart-healthy diet is crucial for maintaining cardiovascular health and reducing the risk of heart disease.

Such a diet focuses on consuming nutrient-rich foods that promote heart health while limiting foods high in unhealthy fats, cholesterol, sodium, and added sugars.

The goal is to maintain a healthy weight, control blood pressure, cholesterol levels, and reduce inflammation.

A key component of a heart-healthy diet is consuming a variety of fruits and vegetables.

These foods are rich in vitamins, minerals, antioxidants, and fiber, which help lower cholesterol, blood pressure, and reduce the risk of heart disease.

Whole grains like oats, brown rice, and whole wheat are also important, providing fiber and nutrients that support heart health.

Lean protein sources such as poultry, fish, legumes, and nuts are essential for a heart-healthy diet. These foods are low in saturated fats and cholesterol, making them good alternatives to red meat, which should be consumed in moderation. Healthy fats from sources like olive oil, avocados, and nuts are beneficial for heart health and should replace saturated and trans fats in the diet.

Limiting sodium intake is crucial for heart health. Processed foods and restaurant meals often contain high levels of sodium, which can increase blood pressure and strain the heart.

Instead, cooking at home using fresh ingredients and herbs and spices to add flavor can help reduce sodium intake.

Finally, staying hydrated with water and limiting sugary beverages is important for heart health. Sugary drinks can contribute to weight gain and increase the risk of heart disease.

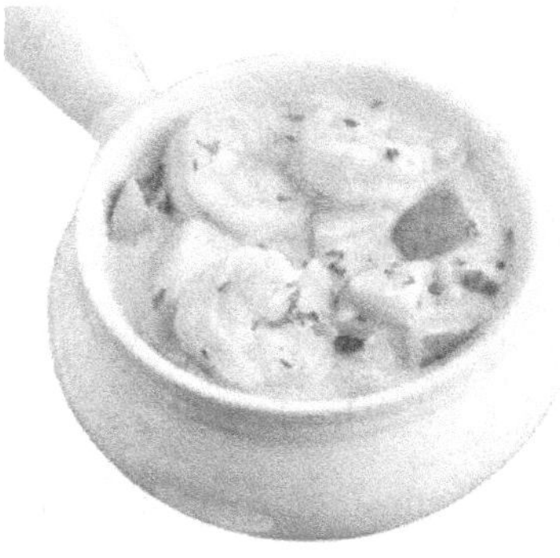

CHAPTER 1

COMMON CAUSES OF HEART ATTACK

1. **Coronary artery disease (CAD):** The most common cause of heart attacks is CAD, where the coronary arteries become narrowed or blocked due to a buildup of cholesterol and other substances, called plaque, on their walls. This reduces blood flow to the heart muscle.

2. **Smoking:** Smoking is a major risk factor for heart attacks. It damages the blood vessels, increases the buildup of plaque, and reduces the oxygen in the blood, all of which can lead to a heart attack.

3. **High blood pressure:** High blood pressure can damage the arteries over time, making them more prone to plaque buildup and narrowing, increasing the risk of a heart attack.

4. **High cholesterol:** High levels of LDL cholesterol (often referred to as "bad" cholesterol) can lead to the buildup of plaque in the arteries, increasing the risk of a heart attack.

5. **Diabetes:** Diabetes increases the risk of heart disease and heart attacks. High blood sugar levels can damage blood vessels and the nerves that control the heart.

6. **Obesity:** Being overweight or obese can lead to other risk factors for heart disease, such as high blood pressure, high cholesterol, and diabetes, increasing the risk of a heart attack.

7. **Family history:** A family history of heart disease can increase the risk of a heart attack, especially if a close relative had a heart attack at an early age.

8. **Physical inactivity:** Lack of regular physical activity is a risk factor for heart disease and can contribute to other risk factors such as obesity, high blood pressure, and high cholesterol.

9. **Stress:** Chronic stress can contribute to heart disease by raising blood pressure and increasing the risk of unhealthy behaviors such as smoking or overeating.

10. **Unhealthy diet:** A diet high in saturated fats, trans fats, cholesterol, and sodium can increase the risk of heart disease and heart attacks.

FOODS TO AVOID FOR SENIORS WITH HEART DISEASES

1. **Saturated and trans fats:** Foods high in saturated and trans fats can raise cholesterol levels and increase the risk of heart disease. These include fatty cuts of meat, full-fat dairy products, butter, lard, and processed foods like cakes, cookies, and fried foods.

2. **Excess salt:** High-sodium foods can increase blood pressure, putting added strain on the heart. Seniors with heart disease should limit their intake of salty foods like processed meats, canned soups, and salty snacks.

3. **Added sugars:** Foods and beverages with added sugars can contribute to weight gain and increase the risk of heart disease. Seniors should avoid sugary drinks, candies, pastries, and other sweets.

4. **Processed and packaged foods:** These often contain high levels of sodium, trans fats, and added sugars, all of which can be detrimental to heart health. Seniors should opt for fresh, whole foods whenever possible.

5. **High-cholesterol foods:** Foods high in cholesterol, such as egg yolks, organ meats, and shellfish, can raise cholesterol levels and increase the risk of heart disease. Seniors should consume these foods in moderation.

6. **Fried foods:** Fried foods are typically high in unhealthy fats and calories, which can contribute to heart disease. Seniors should limit their intake of fried foods and opt for healthier cooking methods like baking, grilling, or steaming.

7. **Alcohol:** Excessive alcohol consumption can raise blood pressure and increase the risk of heart disease. Seniors with heart disease should limit their alcohol intake or avoid it altogether.

8. **Caffeine:** While moderate caffeine consumption is generally safe for most people, excessive intake can cause palpitations and other heart-related issues. Seniors with heart disease should limit their caffeine intake and monitor how it affects them.

9. **Fast food:** Fast food is often high in unhealthy fats, sodium, and calories, all of which can contribute to

heart disease. Seniors should avoid or limit their intake of fast food.

10. **Large meals:** Eating large meals can put strain on the heart and digestive system. Seniors with heart disease should opt for smaller, more frequent meals to reduce the workload on their heart.

DASH DIET AND ITS BENEFITS FOR HEART HEALTH

1. **Emphasis on fruits and vegetables:** The DASH diet encourages the consumption of a variety of fruits and vegetables, which are rich in vitamins, minerals, antioxidants, and fiber. These nutrients help reduce inflammation, lower cholesterol levels, and improve overall heart health.

2. **Whole grains:** The DASH diet emphasizes whole grains like brown rice, whole wheat bread, and oats, which are high in fiber and nutrients. Whole grains can help lower cholesterol levels and reduce the risk of heart disease.

3. **Lean proteins:** The DASH diet recommends lean proteins such as poultry, fish, and legumes, which are

lower in saturated fats compared to red meats. These proteins can help maintain muscle mass and support overall heart health.

4. **Low-fat dairy:** The DASH diet includes low-fat dairy products like milk, yogurt, and cheese, which are good sources of calcium and protein. These foods can help reduce the risk of heart disease, especially when consumed in moderation.

5. **Limited sodium intake:** The DASH diet limits sodium intake to help lower blood pressure and reduce the risk of heart disease. It encourages the use of herbs, spices, and other flavorings to add taste to foods instead of salt.

6. **Reduction of sugary beverages and sweets:** The DASH diet limits the consumption of sugary beverages and sweets, which can contribute to weight gain and increase the risk of heart disease.

7. **Benefits for heart health:** The DASH diet has been shown to lower blood pressure, reduce cholesterol levels, and improve overall heart health. It can also help with weight management, which is important for reducing the risk of heart disease.

8. **Flexibility and sustainability:** The DASH diet is flexible and can be adapted to individual preferences and cultural food choices, making it easier to follow in the long term.

HEALTHY COOKING TECHNIQUES THAT PROMOTE HEART HEALTH

1. **Grilling:** Grilling is a healthy cooking method that allows excess fat to drip off meats, reducing the overall fat content. It also adds a smoky flavor without the need for additional fats.

2. **Baking or roasting:** Baking or roasting foods in the oven with minimal added fats can help retain nutrients while reducing the need for unhealthy oils. Use non-stick pans or line pans with parchment paper to avoid sticking.

3. **Steaming:** Steaming vegetables, fish, and poultry helps retain their nutrients while avoiding the need for added fats. Steaming also helps foods retain their natural flavors.

4. **Broiling:** Broiling food in the oven is similar to grilling, as it allows excess fat to drip away. It's a

quick and easy method for cooking lean meats and vegetables.

5. **Sautéing with healthy fats:** Use heart-healthy oils like olive, avocado, or canola oil for sautéing. Use minimal oil and add vegetables or lean proteins to create flavorful dishes.

6. **Poaching:** Poaching involves cooking food in liquid at a low temperature. It's a healthy cooking method that helps retain moisture and flavor without adding excess fats.

7. **Stir-frying:** Stir-frying quickly cooks vegetables and lean proteins in a small amount of oil over high heat. Use heart-healthy oils and add plenty of vegetables for a nutritious meal.

8. **Using herbs and spices:** Enhance the flavor of your dishes without adding extra salt or unhealthy fats by using herbs, spices, citrus juices, and vinegars.

9. **Reducing salt:** Use salt sparingly and try to replace it with herbs, spices, and other flavorings to enhance the taste of your food without adding extra sodium.

CHAPTER 2

14-DAY MEAL PLAN

DAY 1

Breakfast: Breakfast Burrito

Lunch: Green Goddess Quinoa Bowls with Arugula & Shrimp

Dinner: Morning Burritos with Salsa Verde

DAY 2

Breakfast: Pomegranate Smoothie

Lunch: Grilled Blackened Shrimp Tacos

Dinner: Cauliflower Fried Rice

DAY 3

Breakfast: Overnight Oats

Lunch: Quinoa, Avocado & Chickpea Salad over Mixed Greens

Dinner: Grilled Squash Garlic Bread

DAY 4

Breakfast: Pistachio & Peach Toast

Lunch: Veggie & Hummus Sandwich

Dinner: Pasta with Walnut Pesto and Peas

DAY 5

Breakfast: Blueberry Lemon Oatmeal Parfaits

Lunch: Peach & Spinach Salad with Feta

Dinner: Chicken Salad Collard Wrap

DAY 6

Breakfast: Spinach Omelet Breakfast Sandwich

Lunch: Sichuan Ramen Cup of Noodles with Cabbage & Tofu

Dinner: Butternut Squash and Turmeric Soup

DAY 7

Breakfast: Mango Raspberry Smoothie

Lunch: Stuffed Sweet Potato with Hummus Dressing

Dinner: Baked Chicken Cutlets with Pineapple Rice

DAY 8

Breakfast: Spinach, Peanut Butter & Banana Smoothie

Lunch: Mediterranean Broccoli Pasta Salad

Dinner: Oven-Roasted Salmon with Charred Lemon Vinaigrette

DAY 9

Breakfast: Pineapple-Grapefruit Detox Smoothie

Lunch: Sichuan Ramen Cup of Noodles with Cabbage & Tofu

Dinner: Chicken Kebabs

DAY 10

Breakfast: Oatmeal with Berries and Low-Fat Milk

Lunch: Mixed Greens with Lentils & Sliced Apple

Dinner: Shrimp Scampi with Zoodles

DAY 11

Breakfast: Breakfast Burrito

Lunch: Green Goddess Quinoa Bowls with Arugula & Shrimp

Dinner: Morning Burritos with Salsa Verde

DAY 12

Breakfast: Pomegranate Smoothie

Lunch: Grilled Blackened Shrimp Tacos

Dinner: Cauliflower Fried Rice

DAY 13

Breakfast: Overnight Oats

Lunch: Quinoa, Avocado & Chickpea Salad over Mixed Greens

Dinner: Grilled Squash Garlic Bread

DAY 14

Breakfast: Pistachio & Peach Toast

Lunch: Veggie & Hummus Sandwich

Dinner: Pasta with Walnut Pesto and Peas

CHAPTER 3

NUTRITIOUS RECIPES FOR A HEART HEALTHY DIET

BREAKFAST

Breakfast Burrito

Preparation Time: 15 minutes

Serves: 4

Calories: 350 **Carbs:** 35g **Sodium:** 90mg **Cholesterol:** 80mg **Protein:** 17g **Fat:** 16g

Ingredients:

4 large eggs

1/2 cup diced bell peppers

1/2 cup diced onions

1/2 cup diced tomatoes

1/2 cup cooked black beans

4 whole wheat tortillas

1/2 avocado, sliced

Method of Preparation:

1. In a bowl, beat the eggs.
2. Heat a non-stick skillet over medium heat and add the beaten eggs, bell peppers, onions, and tomatoes.
3. Cook until the eggs are scrambled.
4. Warm the black beans in a separate pot.
5. Place a tortilla on a plate and fill it with the scrambled eggs, black beans, and sliced avocado.
6. Roll it up into a burrito.
7. Repeat for the remaining tortillas.

Pomegranate Smoothie

Preparation Time: 5 minutes

Serves: 1

Calories: 230 **Carbs:** 42g **Sodium:** 70mg **Cholesterol:** 10mg **Protein:** 12g **Fat:** 3g

Ingredients:

1 cup pomegranate seeds

1/2 cup plain Greek yogurt

1/2 cup unsweetened almond milk

1 tablespoon honey

1/2 teaspoon ground cinnamon

Method of Preparation:

1. Combine all ingredients in a blender.
2. Blend until smooth.
3. Pour into a glass and serve.

Overnight Oats

Preparation Time: 5 minutes (plus overnight refrigeration)

Serves: 1

Calories: 250 **Carbs:** 44g **Sodium:** 60mg **Cholesterol:** 0mg **Protein:** 8g **Fat:** 5g

Ingredients:

1/2 cup rolled oats

1/2 cup unsweetened almond milk

1/2 cup diced apples

1 tablespoon chia seeds

1/2 teaspoon ground cinnamon

Method of Preparation:

1. In a jar or container, combine all ingredients.
2. Stir well, cover, and refrigerate overnight.
3. In the morning, stir and enjoy cold or heat in the microwave if desired.

Pistachio & Peach Toast

Preparation Time: 10 minutes

Serves: 2

Calories: 200 **Carbs:** 30g **Sodium:** 100mg **Cholesterol:** 5mg **Protein:** 8g **Fat:** 6g

Ingredients:

2 slices whole grain bread

2 tablespoons low-fat ricotta cheese

1 peach, sliced

1 tablespoon chopped pistachios

1 teaspoon honey (optional)

Method of Preparation:

1. Toast the bread slices until crispy.
2. Spread 1 tablespoon of ricotta cheese on each slice of toast.
3. Top with sliced peaches and chopped pistachios.
4. Drizzle with honey, if desired.

Blueberry Lemon Oatmeal Parfaits

Preparation Time: 10 minutes

Serves: 1

Calories: 300 **Carbs:** 50g **Sodium:** 50mg **Cholesterol:** 5mg **Protein:** 15g **Fat:** 5g

Ingredients:

1 cup cooked steel-cut oats

1/2 cup plain Greek yogurt

1/2 cup blueberries

1 tablespoon honey

1 teaspoon lemon zest

Method of Preparation:

1. In a glass or jar, layer half of the oats, yogurt, and blueberries.
2. Repeat the layers.
3. Drizzle with honey and sprinkle with lemon zest.

Spinach Omelet Breakfast Sandwich

Preparation Time: 15 minutes

Serves: 1

Calories: 400 **Carbs:** 30g **Sodium:** 300mg **Cholesterol:** 370mg **Protein:** 22g **Fat:** 20g

Ingredients:

2 large eggs

1/4 cup chopped spinach

2 slices whole grain bread, toasted

1 slice low-fat cheddar cheese

1/2 avocado, sliced

Method of Preparation:

1. In a bowl, beat the eggs and stir in the chopped spinach.
2. Heat a non-stick skillet over medium heat and pour in the egg mixture.
3. Cook until the eggs are set, then fold in half.
4. Place the omelet on one slice of toasted bread.
5. Top with cheddar cheese, avocado slices, and the other slice of toasted bread.

Mango Raspberry Smoothie

Preparation Time: 5 minutes

Serves: 1

Calories: 250 **Carbs:** 45g **Sodium:** 70mg **Cholesterol:** 5mg **Protein:** 12g **Fat:** 3g

Ingredients:

1 cup frozen mango chunks

1/2 cup frozen raspberries

1/2 cup plain Greek yogurt

1/2 cup unsweetened almond milk

1 tablespoon honey (optional)

Method of Preparation:

1. Combine all ingredients in a blender.
2. Blend until smooth.
3. Pour into a glass and serve.

Spinach, Peanut Butter & Banana Smoothie

Preparation Time: 5 minutes

Serves: 1

Calories: 300 **Carbs:** 35g **Sodium:** 150mg **Cholesterol:** 5mg **Protein:** 15g **Fat:** 12g

Ingredients:

1 banana

1 cup fresh spinach leaves

1 tablespoon natural peanut butter

1/2 cup plain Greek yogurt

1/2 cup unsweetened almond milk

Method of Preparation:

1. Combine all ingredients in a blender.
2. Blend until smooth.
3. Pour into a glass and serve.

Pineapple-Grapefruit Detox Smoothie

Preparation Time: 5 minutes

Serves: 1

Calories: 200 **Carbs:** 40g **Sodium:** 70mg **Cholesterol:** 0mg **Protein:** 5g **Fat:** 3g

Ingredients:

1/2 cup pineapple chunks

1/2 grapefruit, peeled and seeded

1/2 cup coconut water

1/2 teaspoon grated ginger

1 tablespoon chia seeds

Method of Preparation:

1. Combine all ingredients in a blender.
2. Blend until smooth.
3. Pour into a glass and serve.

Oatmeal with Berries and Low-Fat Milk

Preparation Time: 10 minutes

Serves: 1

Calories: 300 **Carbs:** 55g **Sodium:** 120mg **Cholesterol:** 5mg **Protein:** 12g **Fat:** 5g

Ingredients:

1/2 cup rolled oats

1 cup low-fat milk

1/2 cup mixed berries (such as blueberries, strawberries, raspberries)

1 tablespoon honey (optional)

Method of Preparation:

1. In a saucepan, combine the oats and milk.
2. Cook over medium heat, stirring occasionally, until the oats are cooked and the mixture is creamy.
3. Stir in the mixed berries.
4. Remove from heat and let it sit for a few minutes.
5. Drizzle with honey, if desired.

LUNCH

Green Goddess Quinoa Bowls with Arugula & Shrimp

Preparation Time: 30 minutes

Serves: 4

Calories: 400 **Carbs:** 30g **Sodium:** 300mg **Cholesterol:** 150mg **Protein:** 25g **Fat:** 20g

Ingredients:

1 cup quinoa

1 3/4 cups water

1 pound shrimp, peeled and deveined

2 tablespoons olive oil

A pinch of salt and pepper

4 cups arugula

1 avocado, sliced

1/4 cup chopped fresh herbs (such as basil, parsley, chives)

Lemon wedges for serving

Method of Preparation:

1. Rinse the quinoa under cold water.
2. In a saucepan, bring the water to a boil, then add the quinoa. Reduce heat, cover, and simmer for 15-20 minutes until the quinoa is tender and the water is absorbed.
3. In a large skillet, heat olive oil over medium-high heat. Season the shrimp with salt and pepper, then add to the skillet and cook for 2-3 minutes per side until cooked through.
4. Divide the quinoa among bowls, then top with arugula, avocado slices, and cooked shrimp.
5. Sprinkle with chopped herbs and serve with lemon wedges.

Grilled Blackened Shrimp Tacos

Preparation Time: 20 minutes

Serves: 4

Calories: 300 **Carbs:** 30g **Sodium:** 400mg **Cholesterol:** 150mg **Protein:** 25g **Fat:** 10g

Ingredients:

1 pound shrimp, peeled and deveined

1 tablespoon olive oil

1 tablespoon blackening seasoning

8 small corn tortillas

1 cup shredded cabbage

1/2 cup diced tomatoes

1/4 cup chopped cilantro

1/4 cup plain Greek yogurt

Lime wedges for serving

Method of Preparation:

1. Preheat a grill or grill pan over medium-high heat.
2. In a bowl, toss the shrimp with olive oil and blackening seasoning.
3. Grill the shrimp for 2-3 minutes per side until cooked through.
4. Warm the tortillas on the grill for about 30 seconds per side.
5. To assemble the tacos, divide the shrimp among the tortillas, then top with shredded cabbage, diced tomatoes, cilantro, and a dollop of Greek yogurt.
6. Serve with lime wedges.

Quinoa, Avocado & Chickpea Salad over Mixed Greens

Preparation Time: 30 minutes

Serves: 4

Calories: 350 **Carbs:** 50g **Sodium:** 300mg **Cholesterol:** 0mg **Protein:** 12g **Fat:** 15g

Ingredients:

1 cup quinoa

1 3/4 cups water

1 can (15 ounces) chickpeas, drained and rinsed

1 avocado, diced

1/4 cup chopped red onion

1/4 cup chopped fresh cilantro

Juice of 1 lemon

A pinch of salt and pepper

Mixed greens for serving

Method of Preparation:

1. Rinse the quinoa under cold water.
2. In a saucepan, bring the water to a boil, then add the quinoa. Reduce heat, cover, and simmer for 15-20 minutes until the quinoa is tender and the water is absorbed.
3. In a large bowl, combine the cooked quinoa, chickpeas, avocado, red onion, and cilantro.

4. Add lemon juice, salt, and pepper, and toss to combine.

5. Serve the quinoa salad over mixed greens.

Veggie & Hummus Sandwich

Preparation Time: 10 minutes

Serves: 1

Calories: 350 **Carbs:** 45g **Sodium:** 300mg **Cholesterol:** 0mg **Protein:** 10g **Fat:** 15g

Ingredients:

2 slices whole grain bread

2 tablespoons hummus

1/2 cucumber, thinly sliced

1/2 bell pepper, thinly sliced

1/4 red onion, thinly sliced

1/2 avocado, sliced

Handful of spinach leaves

Method of Preparation:

1. Spread hummus evenly on one side of each slice of bread.

2. Layer cucumber slices, bell pepper slices, red onion slices, avocado slices, and spinach leaves on one slice of bread.

3. Top with the other slice of bread to make a sandwich.

Peach & Spinach Salad with Feta

Preparation Time: 10 minutes

Serves: 1

Calories: 250 **Carbs:** 25g **Sodium:** 200mg **Cholesterol:** 15mg **Protein:** 8g **Fat:** 15g

Ingredients:

2 cups fresh spinach leaves

1 peach, sliced

1/4 cup crumbled feta cheese

1 tablespoon balsamic vinegar

1 tablespoon olive oil

Method of Preparation:

1. In a large bowl, combine spinach leaves, peach slices, and feta cheese.
2. In a small bowl, whisk together balsamic vinegar and olive oil.
3. Drizzle the dressing over the salad and toss to combine.

Sichuan Ramen Cup of Noodles with Cabbage & Tofu

Preparation Time: 10 minutes

Serves: 1

Calories: 400 **Carbs:** 45g **Sodium:** 900mg **Cholesterol:** 0mg **Protein:** 15g **Fat:** 18g

Ingredients:

1 package instant ramen noodles (discard seasoning packet)

2 cups water

1 cup shredded cabbage

1/2 block tofu, cubed

2 tablespoons soy sauce

1 tablespoon rice vinegar

1 teaspoon Sichuan peppercorns

Method of Preparation:

1. In a pot, bring the water to a boil.
2. Add the ramen noodles, cabbage, tofu, soy sauce, rice vinegar, and Sichuan peppercorns.
3. Cook for 3-4 minutes until the noodles are tender and the cabbage is wilted.
4. Remove from heat and let it sit for a few minutes before serving.

Vegan Superfood Grain Bowls

Preparation Time: 20 minutes

Serves: 2

Calories: 500 **Carbs:** 60g **Sodium:** 50mg **Cholesterol:** 0mg **Protein:** 20g **Fat:** 20g

Ingredients:

1 cup cooked quinoa

1 cup cooked brown rice

1 cup cooked lentils

1 cup mixed vegetables (such as bell peppers, broccoli, carrots)

1/2 avocado, sliced

1 tablespoon pumpkin seeds

1 tablespoon sunflower seeds

1 tablespoon hemp seeds

2 tablespoons tahini

Method of Preparation:

1. Divide the quinoa, brown rice, lentils, and mixed vegetables among bowls.
2. Top with avocado slices, pumpkin seeds, sunflower seeds, and hemp seeds.
3. Drizzle with tahini before serving.

Stuffed Sweet Potato with Hummus Dressing

Preparation Time: 30 minutes

Serves: 2

Calories: 400 **Carbs:** 70g **Sodium:** 200mg **Cholesterol:** 0mg **Protein:** 10g **Fat:** 10g

Ingredients:

2 medium sweet potatoes

1 cup cooked chickpeas

1/2 red bell pepper, diced

1/4 cup diced red onion

2 tablespoons chopped fresh parsley

1/4 cup hummus

Method of Preparation:

1. Preheat the oven to 400°F (200°C).
2. Prick the sweet potatoes with a fork and bake for 25-30 minutes until tender.
3. In a bowl, mix the chickpeas, bell pepper, red onion, and parsley.
4. Cut the sweet potatoes in half and stuff with the chickpea mixture.
5. Drizzle with hummus before serving.

Mediterranean Broccoli Pasta Salad

Preparation Time: 20 minutes

Serves: 4

Calories: 350 **Carbs:** 50g **Sodium:** 300mg **Cholesterol:** 5mg **Protein:** 12g **Fat:** 12g

Ingredients:

8 oz whole wheat pasta

2 cups broccoli florets

1/2 cup diced red onion

1/2 cup diced cucumber

1/2 cup halved cherry tomatoes

1/4 cup chopped Kalamata olives

1/4 cup crumbled feta cheese

2 tablespoons olive oil

2 tablespoons lemon juice

1 teaspoon dried oregano

Method of Preparation:

1. Cook the pasta according to package instructions, adding the broccoli to the boiling water in the last 2 minutes of cooking.
2. Drain the pasta and broccoli and rinse with cold water.
3. In a large bowl, combine the pasta, broccoli, red onion, cucumber, tomatoes, olives, and feta cheese.
4. In a small bowl, whisk together the olive oil, lemon juice, and oregano. Pour over the pasta salad and toss to combine.

Mixed Greens with Lentils & Sliced Apple

Preparation Time: 15 minutes

Serves: 2

Calories: 300 **Carbs:** 40g **Sodium:** 50mg **Cholesterol:** 0mg **Protein:** 12g **Fat:** 10g

Ingredients:

4 cups mixed greens

1 cup cooked lentils

1 apple, thinly sliced

1/4 cup chopped walnuts

2 tablespoons balsamic vinegar

1 tablespoon olive oil

Method of Preparation:

1. In a large bowl, combine the mixed greens, cooked lentils, apple slices, and chopped walnuts.
2. In a small bowl, whisk together the balsamic vinegar and olive oil.
3. Pour over the salad and toss to combine.

DINNER

Morning Burritos with Salsa Verde

Preparation Time: 15 minutes

Serves: 4

Calories: 300 **Carbs:** 35g **Sodium:** 400mg **Cholesterol:** 170mg **Protein:** 15g **Fat:** 10g

Ingredients:

4 whole wheat tortillas

4 large eggs

1 cup black beans, drained and rinsed

1/2 cup shredded low-fat cheese

1/2 cup salsa Verde

1/4 cup chopped fresh cilantro

Method of Preparation:

1. In a skillet, scramble the eggs over medium heat.
2. Warm the tortillas in the skillet or microwave.
3. Divide the scrambled eggs, black beans, cheese, and salsa Verde among the tortillas.
4. Sprinkle with chopped cilantro.
5. Roll up the tortillas and serve.

Cauliflower Fried Rice

Preparation Time: 20 minutes

Serves: 4

Calories: 150 **Carbs:** 15g **Sodium:** 300mg **Cholesterol:** 0mg **Protein:** 5g **Fat:** 8g

Ingredients:

1 small head cauliflower, grated

1 tablespoon olive oil

2 cloves garlic, minced

1/2 cup diced carrots

1/2 cup frozen peas

2 green onions, chopped

2 tablespoons low-sodium soy sauce

1 tablespoon sesame oil

Method of Preparation:

1. In a large skillet, heat olive oil over medium heat.
2. Add garlic and cook for 1 minute.
3. Add grated cauliflower, carrots, peas, and green onions.
4. Cook for 5-7 minutes, stirring occasionally.
5. Stir in soy sauce and sesame oil.

6. Cook for an additional 2-3 minutes, then serve.

Grilled Squash Garlic Bread

Preparation Time: 15 minutes

Serves: 4

Calories: 200 **Carbs:** 25g **Sodium:** 250mg **Cholesterol:** 5mg **Protein:** 8g **Fat:** 8g

Ingredients:

1 small yellow squash, sliced

1 small zucchini, sliced

1 tablespoon olive oil

4 slices whole grain bread

2 cloves garlic, minced

1/4 cup grated Parmesan cheese

Method of Preparation:

1. Preheat a grill or grill pan over medium-high heat.
2. Toss the squash and zucchini slices with olive oil.

3. Grill the squash and zucchini for 3-4 minutes per side until tender.

4. Toast the bread slices on the grill.

5. Rub the toasted bread with minced garlic.

6. Top each slice of bread with grilled squash and zucchini.

7. Sprinkle with Parmesan cheese before serving.

Pasta with Walnut Pesto and Peas

Preparation Time: 20 minutes

Serves: 4

Calories: 400 **Carbs:** 45g **Sodium:** 150mg **Cholesterol:** 5mg **Protein:** 12g **Fat:** 20g

Ingredients:

8 oz whole wheat pasta

1/2 cup walnuts

2 cups fresh basil leaves

2 cloves garlic

1/4 cup grated Parmesan cheese

1/4 cup olive oil

1 cup frozen peas, thawed

Method of Preparation:

1. Cook the pasta according to package instructions.
2. In a food processor, combine walnuts, basil, garlic, and Parmesan cheese.
3. Pulse until finely chopped.
4. With the processor running, slowly add olive oil until the mixture forms a paste.
5. Toss the cooked pasta with the pesto and peas.

Chicken Salad Collard Wrap

Preparation Time: 15 minutes

Serves: 4

Calories: 250 **Carbs:** 15g **Sodium:** 200mg **Cholesterol:** 50mg **Protein:** 25g **Fat:** 10g

Ingredients:

2 cups cooked chicken breast, diced

1/4 cup plain Greek yogurt

1 tablespoon Dijon mustard

1/4 cup chopped celery

1/4 cup chopped red onion

1/4 cup dried cranberries

4 large collard green leaves

Method of Preparation:

1. In a bowl, combine chicken, Greek yogurt, Dijon mustard, celery, red onion, and dried cranberries. Mix well.
2. Lay a collard green leaf flat on a cutting board. Remove the tough stem.
3. Spoon some of the chicken salad onto the collard green leaf and wrap it up like a burrito.

Butternut Squash and Turmeric Soup

Preparation Time: 30 minutes

Serves: 4

Calories: 200 **Carbs:** 30g **Sodium:** 600mg **Cholesterol:** 0mg **Protein:** 5g **Fat:** 8g

Ingredients:

1 butternut squash, peeled, seeded, and cubed

1 onion, chopped

2 cloves garlic, minced

1 tablespoon olive oil

4 cups vegetable broth

1 teaspoon ground turmeric

A pinch of salt and pepper

Method of Preparation:

1. In a large pot, heat olive oil over medium heat.
2. Add onion and garlic and cook until softened.
3. Add butternut squash, vegetable broth, turmeric, salt, and pepper.
4. Bring to a boil, then reduce heat and simmer for 20-25 minutes until the squash is tender.
5. Use an immersion blender to blend the soup until smooth.

Baked Chicken Cutlets with Pineapple Rice

Preparation Time: 30 minutes

Serves: 4

Calories: 350 **Carbs:** 40g **Sodium:** 300mg **Cholesterol:** 70mg **Protein:** 30g **Fat:** 8g

Ingredients:

4 boneless, skinless chicken breast cutlets

1/2 cup whole wheat breadcrumbs

1/4 cup grated Parmesan cheese

1 teaspoon Italian seasoning

1/2 cup pineapple juice

2 cups cooked brown rice

1 cup diced pineapple

Method of Preparation:

1. Preheat oven to 400°F (200°C).

2. In a bowl, combine breadcrumbs, Parmesan cheese, and Italian seasoning.

3. Dip each chicken cutlet in pineapple juice, then coat with breadcrumb mixture.

4. Place the chicken on a baking sheet and bake for 20-25 minutes until cooked through.

5. In a separate bowl, combine cooked brown rice and diced pineapple.

6. Serve the chicken cutlets with the pineapple rice.

Oven-Roasted Salmon with Charred Lemon Vinaigrette

Preparation Time: 20 minutes

Serves: 4

Calories: 300 **Carbs:** 10g **Sodium:** 200mg **Cholesterol:** 80mg **Protein:** 30g **Fat:** 15g

Ingredients:

4 salmon fillets

A pinch of salt and pepper

2 lemons, halved

2 tablespoons olive oil

1 tablespoon honey

1 tablespoon Dijon mustard

1 clove garlic, minced

2 tablespoons chopped fresh parsley

Method of Preparation:

1. Preheat the oven to 400°F (200°C).
2. Season the salmon fillets with salt and pepper and place them on a baking sheet.
3. Place the lemon halves cut side down on the baking sheet.
4. Roast in the oven for 12-15 minutes until the salmon is cooked through.
5. In a small bowl, whisk together olive oil, honey, mustard, garlic, and parsley.
6. Squeeze the roasted lemons into the dressing and whisk to combine.
7. Serve the salmon with the charred lemon vinaigrette.

Chicken Kebabs

Preparation Time: 25 minutes

Serves: 4

Calories: 250 **Carbs:** 10g **Sodium:** 100mg **Cholesterol:** 70mg **Protein:** 25g **Fat:** 12g

Ingredients:

1 lb. boneless, skinless chicken breasts, cut into cubes

1 bell pepper, cut into chunks

1 onion, cut into chunks

1 zucchini, sliced

1/4 cup olive oil

2 tablespoons lemon juice

2 cloves garlic, minced

1 teaspoon dried oregano

Method of Preparation:

1. In a bowl, combine olive oil, lemon juice, garlic, and oregano.

2. Add chicken cubes and vegetables to the bowl and toss to coat.

3. Thread chicken and vegetables onto skewers.

4. Grill kebabs over medium heat for 10-15 minutes, turning occasionally, until chicken is cooked through.

Shrimp Scampi with Zoodles

Preparation Time: 20 minutes

Serves: 4

Calories: 200 **Carbs:** 10g **Sodium:** 200mg **Cholesterol:** 150mg **Protein:** 25g **Fat:** 8g

Ingredients:

1 lb. shrimp, peeled and deveined

2 tablespoons olive oil

4 cloves garlic, minced

1/2 cup low-sodium chicken broth

1/4 cup white wine

2 tablespoons lemon juice

4 zucchinis, spiralized into noodles

2 tablespoons chopped fresh parsley

Method of Preparation:

1. In a large skillet, heat olive oil over medium heat.
2. Add garlic and cook for 1 minute.
3. Add shrimp and cook for 2-3 minutes until pink.
4. Remove shrimp from the skillet and set aside.
5. Add chicken broth, white wine, and lemon juice to the skillet. Bring to a simmer.
6. Add zucchini noodles and cook for 2-3 minutes until tender.
7. Return shrimp to the skillet and toss to combine.
8. Sprinkle with chopped parsley before serving.

SEAFOOD MAINS

Seafood Chowder

Preparation Time: 30 minutes

Serves: 4

Calories: 300 **Carbs:** 25g **Sodium:** 400mg **Cholesterol:** 150mg **Protein:** 30g **Fat:** 8g

Ingredients:

1 tablespoon olive oil

1 onion, chopped

2 stalks celery, chopped

2 carrots, chopped

2 cloves garlic, minced

4 cups low-sodium chicken broth

1 cup diced potatoes

1 teaspoon dried thyme

1/2 teaspoon smoked paprika

1/2 lb. white fish fillets, cubed

1/2 lb. shrimp, peeled and deveined

1 cup low-fat milk

A pinch of salt and pepper

Method of Preparation:

1. In a large pot, heat olive oil over medium heat.

2. Add onion, celery, carrots, and garlic.

3. Cook until vegetables are softened.

4. Add chicken broth, potatoes, thyme, and smoked paprika.

5. Bring to a simmer and cook until potatoes are tender.

6. Add fish and shrimp.

7. Cook for 5-7 minutes until seafood is cooked through.

8. Stir in milk and season with salt and pepper.

9. Serve hot.

Fish with Moroccan Lentil Salad

Preparation Time: 25 minutes

Serves: 4

Calories: 250 **Carbs:** 15g **Sodium:** 100mg **Cholesterol:** 50mg **Protein:** 25g **Fat:** 10g

Ingredients:

4 white fish fillets

1 tablespoon olive oil

1 teaspoon ground cumin

1/2 teaspoon ground cinnamon

1/2 teaspoon ground coriander

1/2 cup cooked lentils

1/4 cup chopped fresh parsley

1/4 cup chopped fresh mint

1/4 cup chopped red onion

1/4 cup chopped cucumber

1/4 cup chopped red bell pepper

2 tablespoons lemon juice

Method of Preparation:

1. Preheat the oven to 400°F (200°C).
2. Rub the fish fillets with olive oil, cumin, cinnamon, and coriander.
3. Place the fish on a baking sheet and bake for 15-20 minutes until cooked through.
4. In a bowl, combine cooked lentils, parsley, mint, red onion, cucumber, red bell pepper, and lemon juice.
5. Serve the fish with the lentil salad.

Lemon-Garlic Salmon Bites

Preparation Time: 15 minutes

Serves: 4

Calories: 200 **Carbs:** 1g **Sodium:** 100mg **Cholesterol:** 60mg **Protein:** 25g **Fat:** 10g

Ingredients:

1 lb. salmon fillet, cut into bite-sized pieces

2 tablespoons olive oil

2 cloves garlic, minced

Zest of 1 lemon

Juice of 1 lemon

A pinch of salt and pepper

Method of Preparation:

1. Preheat the oven to 400°F (200°C).
2. In a bowl, combine salmon, olive oil, garlic, lemon zest, lemon juice, salt, and pepper.
3. Spread the salmon pieces on a baking sheet.

4. Bake for 10-12 minutes until salmon is cooked through.

Salmon Tikka Parcels with Rice Salad

Preparation Time: 30 minutes

Serves: 4

Calories: 350 **Carbs:** 30g **Sodium:** 200mg **Cholesterol:** 80mg **Protein:** 30g **Fat:** 12g

Ingredients:

4 salmon fillets

1/2 cup plain Greek yogurt

2 tablespoons tikka masala paste

1 teaspoon ground cumin

1 teaspoon ground coriander

1 teaspoon smoked paprika

1 cup cooked brown rice

1/4 cup chopped fresh cilantro

1/4 cup chopped fresh mint

1/4 cup chopped red onion

1/4 cup chopped cucumber

1/4 cup chopped red bell pepper

2 tablespoons lemon juice

Method of Preparation:

1. Preheat the oven to 400°F (200°C).
2. In a bowl, combine yogurt, tikka masala pastes, cumin, coriander, and smoked paprika.
3. Spread the yogurt mixture over the salmon fillets.
4. Wrap each salmon fillet in aluminum foil and place on a baking sheet.
5. Bake for 15-20 minutes until salmon is cooked through.
6. In a bowl, combine cooked brown rice, cilantro, mint, red onion, cucumber, red bell pepper, and lemon juice.
7. Serve the salmon parcels with the rice salad.

Italian Fish Parcels

Preparation Time: 20 minutes

Serves: 4

Calories: 200 **Carbs:** 5g **Sodium:** 200mg **Cholesterol:** 50mg **Protein:** 25g **Fat:** 8g

Ingredients:

4 white fish fillets

1 tablespoon olive oil

1/2 cup cherry tomatoes, halved

1/4 cup sliced black olives

2 tablespoons chopped fresh basil

2 tablespoons chopped fresh parsley

2 tablespoons lemon juice

Method of Preparation:

1. Preheat the oven to 400°F (200°C).
2. Place each fish fillet on a piece of aluminum foil.

3. Drizzle with olive oil and sprinkle with cherry tomatoes, black olives, basil, parsley, and lemon juice.

4. Fold the aluminum foil to form parcels.

5. Bake for 15-20 minutes until fish is cooked through.

SOUPS AND STEWS

Slow-Cooker Chicken & White Bean Stew

Preparation Time: 15 minutes

Serves: 6

Calories: 320 **Carbs:** 35g **Sodium:** 80mg **Cholesterol:** 45mg **Protein:** 30g **Fat:** 5g

Ingredients:

1 lb. boneless, skinless chicken breasts, diced

2 cans (15 oz each) low-sodium white beans, drained and rinsed

1 onion, chopped

2 carrots, chopped

2 celery stalks, chopped

3 cloves garlic, minced

1 teaspoon dried thyme

1 teaspoon dried rosemary

4 cups low-sodium chicken broth

2 cups water

A pinch of salt and pepper

Fresh parsley, chopped (optional, for garnish)

Method of Preparation:

1. In a slow cooker, combine chicken, white beans, onion, carrots, celery, garlic, thyme, rosemary, chicken broth, and water.
2. Cook on low for 6-8 hours or on high for 3-4 hours, until chicken is cooked through and vegetables are tender.
3. Season with A pinch of salt and pepper. Garnish with fresh parsley before serving, if desired.

Cream of Turkey & Wild Rice Soup

Preparation Time: 10 minutes

Serves: 6

Calories: 280 **Carbs:** 30g **Sodium:** 90mg **Cholesterol:** 50mg **Protein:** 25g **Fat:** 4g

Ingredients:

1 lb. turkey breast, diced

1 cup wild rice

1 onion, chopped

2 carrots, chopped

2 celery stalks, chopped

3 cloves garlic, minced

4 cups low-sodium chicken broth

2 cups water

1 teaspoon dried thyme

A pinch of salt and pepper

Fresh parsley, chopped (optional, for garnish)

Method of Preparation:

1. In a large pot, combine turkey breast, wild rice, onion, carrots, celery, garlic, chicken broth, water, and thyme.
2. Bring to a boil, then reduce heat and simmer for 20-25 minutes, until turkey is cooked through and rice is tender.
3. Season with A pinch of salt and pepper. Garnish with fresh parsley before serving, if desired.

Four-Bean & Pumpkin Chili

Preparation Time: 15 minutes

Serves: 6

Calories: 320 **Carbs:** 55g **Sodium:** 60mg **Cholesterol:** 0mg **Protein:** 15g **Fat:** 2g

Ingredients:

1 can (15 oz) low-sodium black beans, drained and rinsed

1 can (15 oz) low-sodium kidney beans, drained and rinsed

1 can (15 oz) low-sodium pinto beans, drained and rinsed

1 can (15 oz) low-sodium garbanzo beans, drained and rinsed

1 can (15 oz) pumpkin puree

1 onion, chopped

1 bell pepper, chopped

2 cloves garlic, minced

1 tablespoon chili powder

1 teaspoon cumin

4 cups low-sodium vegetable broth

A pinch of salt and pepper

Fresh cilantro, chopped (optional, for garnish)

Method of Preparation:

1. In a large pot, combine black beans, kidney beans, pinto beans, garbanzo beans, pumpkin puree, onion, bell pepper, garlic, chili powder, cumin, and vegetable broth.

2. Bring to a boil, then reduce heat and simmer for 20-25 minutes, stirring occasionally.

3. Season with A pinch of salt and pepper. Garnish with fresh cilantro before serving, if desired.

Grilled Tomato Gazpacho

Preparation Time: 20 minutes

Serves: 6

Calories: 150 **Carbs:** 15g **Sodium:** 70mg **Cholesterol:** 0mg **Protein:** 2g **Fat:** 10g

Ingredients:

2 lbs. tomatoes, halved

1 cucumber, peeled and chopped

1 bell pepper, chopped

1 onion, chopped

2 cloves garlic, minced

1/4 cup olive oil

2 tablespoons red wine vinegar

1 teaspoon dried oregano

A pinch of salt and pepper

Fresh basil, chopped (optional, for garnish)

Method of Preparation:

1. Preheat grill to medium-high heat.
2. Place tomatoes on grill, cut side down, and grill for 5-7 minutes, until slightly charred.
3. In a blender, combine grilled tomatoes, cucumber, bell pepper, onion, garlic, olive oil, red wine vinegar, oregano, salt, and pepper. Blend until smooth.
4. Chill in the refrigerator for at least 1 hour before serving.
5. Garnish with fresh basil before serving, if desired.

Chicken & White Bean Soup

Preparation Time: 15 minutes

Serves: 6

Calories: 300 **Carbs:** 30g **Sodium:** 90mg **Cholesterol:** 55mg **Protein:** 25g **Fat:** 4g

Ingredients:

1 lb. boneless, skinless chicken thighs, diced

2 cans (15 oz each) low-sodium white beans, drained and rinsed

1 onion, chopped

2 carrots, chopped

2 celery stalks, chopped

3 cloves garlic, minced

1 teaspoon dried thyme

1 teaspoon dried rosemary

4 cups low-sodium chicken broth

2 cups water

A pinch of salt and pepper

Fresh parsley, chopped (optional, for garnish)

Method of Preparation:

1. In a large pot, combine chicken thighs, white beans, onion, carrots, celery, garlic, thyme, rosemary, chicken broth, and water.

2. Bring to a boil, then reduce heat and simmer for 20-25 minutes, until chicken is cooked through and vegetables are tender.

3. Season with A pinch of salt and pepper. Garnish with fresh parsley before serving, if desired.

POULTRY MAINS

Creamy White Chili with Cream Cheese

Preparation Time: 20 minutes

Serves: 6

Calories: 350 **Carbs:** 30g **Sodium:** 90mg **Cholesterol:** 60mg **Protein:** 30g **Fat:** 10g

Ingredients:

1 lb. boneless, skinless chicken breasts, diced

2 cans (15 oz each) white beans, drained and rinsed

1 onion, chopped

2 cloves garlic, minced

1 can (4 oz) diced green chilies

4 cups low-sodium chicken broth

1 teaspoon cumin

1/2 teaspoon oregano

1/2 teaspoon chili powder

A pinch of salt and pepper

4 oz cream cheese, softened

Fresh cilantro, chopped (optional, for garnish)

Method of Preparation:

1. In a large pot, combine chicken, white beans, onion, garlic, green chilies, chicken broth, cumin, oregano, chili powder, salt, and pepper.
2. Bring to a boil, then reduce heat and simmer for 15-20 minutes, until chicken is cooked through.
3. Stir in cream cheese until melted and well combined.

4. Garnish with fresh cilantro before serving, if desired.

Creamy Chicken, Brussels Sprouts & Mushrooms

Preparation Time: 25 minutes

Serves: 4

Calories: 300 **Carbs:** 20g **Sodium:** 80mg **Cholesterol:** 70mg **Protein:** 30g **Fat:** 10g

Ingredients:

1 lb. boneless, skinless chicken thighs, diced

1 lb. Brussels sprouts, halved

8 oz mushrooms, sliced

1 onion, chopped

2 cloves garlic, minced

1 cup low-sodium chicken broth

1/2 cup plain Greek yogurt

1 tablespoon Dijon mustard

1 tablespoon olive oil

A pinch of salt and pepper

Fresh parsley, chopped (optional, for garnish)

Metho of Preparation:

1. In a large skillet, heat olive oil over medium heat.
2. Add chicken thighs and cook until browned, about 5 minutes.
3. Add Brussels sprouts, mushrooms, onion, and garlic to the skillet.
4. Cook for another 5 minutes, until vegetables are tender.
5. Stir in chicken broth, Greek yogurt, and Dijon mustard. Simmer for 5 minutes, until sauce is creamy and chicken is cooked through.
6. Season with A pinch of salt and pepper.
7. Garnish with fresh parsley before serving, if desired.

Roasted Chicken Thighs with Sweet Potato Wedges and Brussels Sprouts

Preparation Time: 25 minutes

Serves: 4

Calories: 350 **Carbs:** 30g **Sodium:** 70mg **Cholesterol:** 80mg **Protein:** 30g **Fat:** 12g

Ingredients:

1 lb. chicken thighs

2 sweet potatoes, cut into wedges

1 lb. Brussels sprouts, halved

2 tablespoons olive oil

1 teaspoon paprika

1/2 teaspoon garlic powder

A pinch of salt and pepper

Fresh thyme, chopped (optional, for garnish)

Method of Preparation:

1. Preheat oven to 425°F (220°C).
2. In a large bowl, combine chicken thighs, sweet potato wedges, Brussels sprouts, olive oil, paprika, garlic powder, salt, and pepper. Toss to coat.
3. Spread mixture on a baking sheet in a single layer.

4. Roast in the preheated oven for 25-30 minutes, until chicken is cooked through and vegetables are tender.

5. Garnish with fresh thyme before serving, if desired.

Ranch Chicken and Vegetables

Preparation Time: 25 minutes

Serves: 4

Calories: 320 **Carbs:** 30g **Sodium:** 80mg **Cholesterol:** 70mg **Protein:** 30g **Fat:** 10g

Ingredients:

1 lb. chicken breasts, diced

1 lb. baby potatoes, halved

1 lb. green beans, trimmed

1/2 cup ranch dressing (low-fat)

1 tablespoon olive oil

1 teaspoon garlic powder

A pinch of salt and pepper

Fresh dill, chopped (optional, for garnish)

Method of Preparation:

1. Preheat oven to 400°F (200°C).
2. In a large bowl, combine chicken breasts, baby potatoes, green beans, ranch dressing, olive oil, garlic powder, salt, and pepper. Toss to coat.
3. Spread mixture on a baking sheet in a single layer.
4. Roast in the preheated oven for 25-30 minutes, until chicken is cooked through and vegetables are tender.
5. Garnish with fresh dill before serving, if desired.

Chipotle Turkey Quinoa Burrito Bowl

Preparation Time: 25 minutes

Serves: 6

Calories: 330 **Carbs:** 40g **Sodium:** 90mg **Cholesterol:** 60mg **Protein:** 25g **Fat:** 8g

Ingredients:

1 lb. ground turkey

1 cup quinoa, rinsed

1 can (15 oz) black beans, drained and rinsed

1 bell pepper, chopped

1 onion, chopped

2 cloves garlic, minced

1 teaspoon chipotle powder

1 teaspoon cumin

2 cups low-sodium chicken broth

A pinch of salt and pepper

Fresh cilantro, chopped (optional, for garnish)

Method of Preparation:

1. In a large skillet, cook ground turkey over medium heat until browned, breaking it up with a spoon.
2. Add quinoa, black beans, bell pepper, onion, garlic, chipotle powder, cumin, chicken broth, salt, and pepper to the skillet. Stir to combine.
3. Bring to a boil, then reduce heat and simmer for 15-20 minutes, until quinoa is cooked and liquid is absorbed.
4. Garnish with fresh cilantro before serving, if desired.

2-Bite Mini Pumpkin Cheesecake Tarts

Preparation Time: 15 minutes

Serves: 12

Calories: 60 **Carbs:** 6g **Sodium:** 40mg **Cholesterol:** 5mg **Protein:** 1g **Fat:** 3g

Ingredients:

8 oz reduced-fat cream cheese, softened

1/2 cup canned pumpkin puree

1/4 cup stevia

1 teaspoon pumpkin pie spice

24 mini phyllo shells

Method of Preparation:

1. In a bowl, beat cream cheese, pumpkin, sugar, and pumpkin pie spice until smooth.
2. Spoon mixture into phyllo shells.

3. Refrigerate until serving.

Low-Sugar Strawberry Rhubarb Crisp

Preparation Time: 20 minutes

Serves: 6

Calories: 120 **Carbs:** 20g **Sodium:** 0mg **Cholesterol:** 5mg

Protein: 2g **Fat:** 4g

Ingredients:

2 cups sliced strawberries

2 cups sliced rhubarb

1/4 cup stevia

1/2 cup old-fashioned oats

1/4 cup whole wheat flour

1/4 cup chopped walnuts

2 tablespoons butter, melted

1/2 teaspoon cinnamon

Method of Preparation:

1. Preheat oven to 350°F (175°C).
2. In a bowl, combine strawberries, rhubarb, and sugar. Spread in a baking dish.
3. In another bowl, combine oats, flour, walnuts, butter, and cinnamon. Sprinkle over fruit.
4. Bake for 25-30 minutes, until fruit is bubbly and topping is golden.

Mbatata (Sweet Potato Cookies)

Preparation Time: 25 minutes

Serves: 24

Calories: 120 **Carbs:** 20g **Sodium:** 90mg **Cholesterol:** 10mg **Protein:** 2g **Fat:** 4g

Ingredients:

2 cups mashed sweet potatoes

1/2 cup stevia

1/4 cup butter, melted

1 teaspoon vanilla extract

1/2 cup whole wheat flour

1/2 teaspoon baking powder

1/2 teaspoon cinnamon

1/4 teaspoon nutmeg

1/4 teaspoon salt

1/4 cup chopped walnuts (optional)

Method of Preparation:

1. Preheat oven to 350°F (175°C).
2. Line a baking sheet with parchment paper.
3. In a bowl, combine sweet potatoes, stevia, butter, and vanilla.
4. In another bowl, combine flour, baking powder, cinnamon, nutmeg, and salt.
5. Stir into sweet potato mixture.
6. Fold in walnuts, if using.
7. Drop by tablespoonfuls onto prepared baking sheet. Flatten slightly.
8. Bake for 15-20 minutes, until cookies are set and lightly browned.

Banana Bran Muffin

Preparation Time: 20 minutes

Serves: 12

Calories: 80 **Carbs:** 18g **Sodium:** 120mg **Cholesterol:** 15mg **Protein:** 2g **Fat:** 1g

Ingredients:

1 cup whole wheat flour

1/2 cup wheat bran

1/4 cup stevia

1 teaspoon baking powder

1/2 teaspoon baking soda

1/4 teaspoon salt

2 ripe bananas, mashed

1/4 cup low-fat milk

1/4 cup unsweetened applesauce

1 egg

Method of Preparation:

1. Preheat oven to 350°F (175°C).
2. Line a muffin tin with paper liners.
3. In a bowl, combine flour, wheat bran, stevia, baking powder, baking soda, and salt.
4. In another bowl, combine bananas, milk, applesauce, and egg.
5. Stir into dry ingredients just until moistened.
6. Spoon batter into muffin cups.
7. Bake for 15-18 minutes, until a toothpick inserted into the center comes out clean.

Apple Crumble with Oats

Preparation Time: 20 minutes

Serves: 6

Calories: 120 **Carbs:** 25g **Sodium:** 0mg **Cholesterol:** 5mg **Protein:** 1g **Fat:** 3g

Ingredients:

4 cups sliced apples

1/2 cup old-fashioned oats

1/4 cup whole wheat flour

1/4 cup stevia

1/2 teaspoon cinnamon

2 tablespoons butter, melted

Method of Preparation:

1. Preheat oven to 350°F (175°C).
2. Lightly grease a baking dish.
3. Spread apples in the baking dish.
4. In a bowl, combine oats, flour, stevia, cinnamon, and butter.
5. Sprinkle over apples.
6. Bake for 25-30 minutes, until apples are tender and topping is golden.

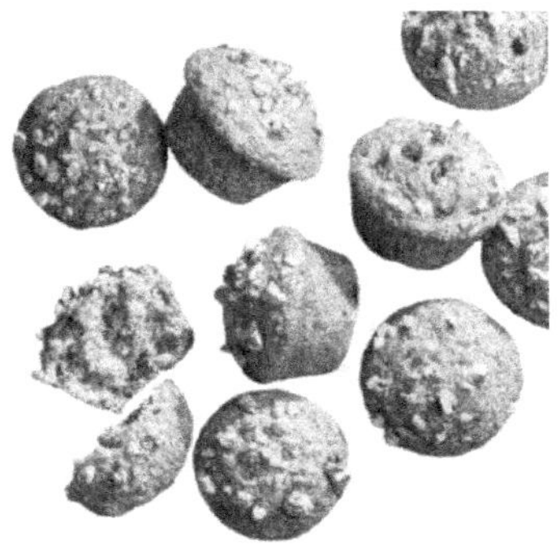

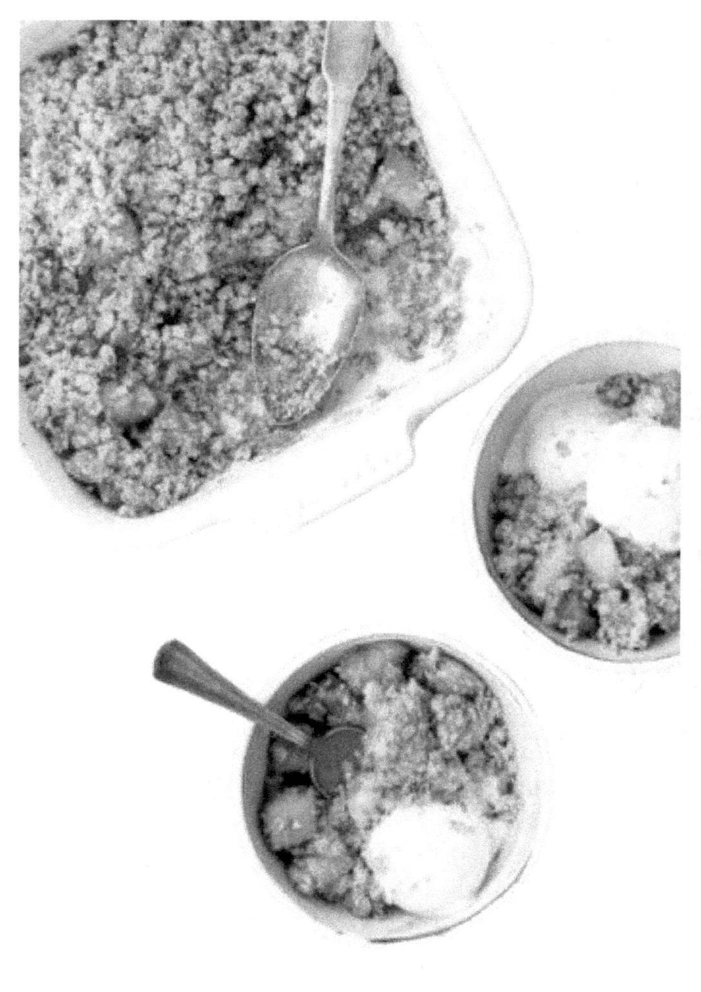

CONCLUSION

In conclusion, maintaining heart health is crucial for overall well-being, and diet plays a significant role in achieving this goal.

The DASH diet, with its emphasis on fruits, vegetables, whole grains, lean proteins, and low-fat dairy, is a valuable tool for promoting heart health and reducing the risk of heart disease.

By following the principles of the DASH diet and incorporating healthy cooking techniques into meal preparation, you can improve your heart health and overall quality of life.

Healthy cooking techniques such as grilling, baking, steaming, and sautéing with healthy fats can help reduce the intake of unhealthy fats, sodium, and calories while retaining the nutritional value and flavor of foods.

Using herbs, spices, and other flavorings instead of salt can also enhance the taste of dishes without adding extra sodium.

It's important to note that while diet and cooking techniques are important for heart health, they should be part of a comprehensive approach that includes regular physical activity, maintaining a healthy weight, and avoiding smoking.

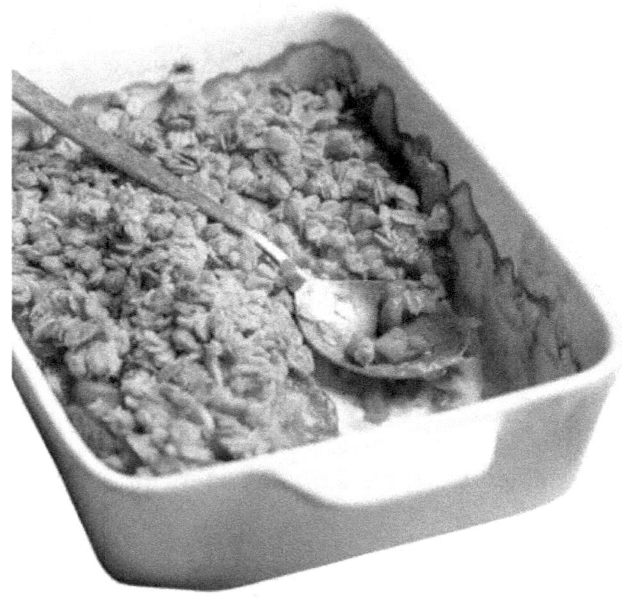

www.ingramcontent.com/pod-product-compliance
Lightning Source LLC
Chambersburg PA
CBHW050818250726
48653CB00006B/2291